"The Women's Guide To Burning Fat & Building Muscle"
By Tony Xhudo M.S., H.N.
Board Certified by A.A.D.P.

The Women's Guide to Burning Fat & Building Muscle
By Tony Xhudo M.S., H.N., Board Certified by A. A. D. P.
Published by Dawn Xhudo
Copyright 2012 Dawn Xhudo

Disclaimer

DISCLAIMER: This information was gathered from sources including textbooks, and reports. Neither the author nor publisher assumes any liability for the information presented in this text. This book is not intended to provide medical advice. The purpose of this reference book is only to provide a compendium of information for the reader, for entertainment purposes only. Readers should consult with appropriate medical authorities before using any related products and the proper legal authorities if unsure of the status of substances described herein.

Disclosure

Other Books by Author Tony Xhudo M.S., H.N.

- ⅄ **How to Build Muscle in Your Advanced Years**

- ⅄ **The Ultimate Guide to Enhancing Your Sex Life**

- ⅄ **The Everyday Guy's Guide to getting & having More Sex**

- ⅄ **Smart Nutrients for Smart Babies**

- ⅄ **The Secrets of gaining Mass Muscle Made Easy**

- ⅄ **The Anabolic Edge to Mass Muscle**

- ⅄ **Ergogenic Aids for Bodybuilding**

- ⅄ **Natural Gh Releasers "The Fountain of Youth"**

- ⅄ **How to Lower Your Cholesterol Without Drugs**

- ⅄ **Holistic Therapy For Fibromyalgia The Cause & The Remedy**

- ⅄ **The Fat Ass Guide to Losing Weight**

- ⅄ **Aphrodisiacs: Prove Sex Boosters That Work**

TABLE OF CONTENTS

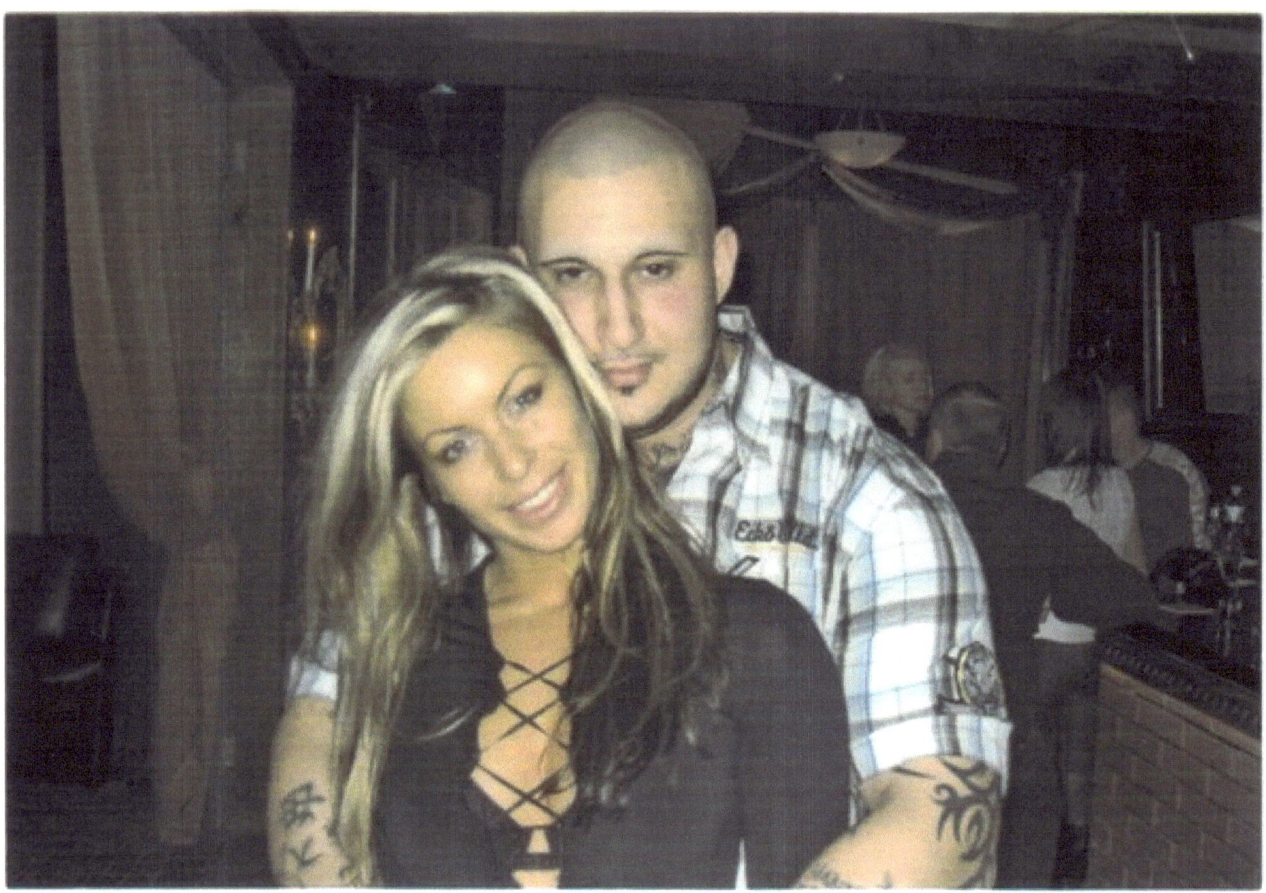

Dedication

I would like to thank my daughter-in-law, Alexandria Xhudo. Our new fitness model for her efforts in following the routines and nutritional guide lines that were addressed in this publication. With a special thanks to our son, A.J. Xhudo who also was a personal health and muscle project since he was 10 years old that has graced the cover on our earlier publication in "The Secrets Of Muscle Mass Made Easy". I love you'se both for always being there for "Bobby"

I would also like to bestow my love and appreciation to a special person in my life, Dawn Xhudo, my lovely wife that has helped me in publishing many of my books. For without her help and devotion, it would not have been possible !

Introduction

I know that there many women out there that do want to look just as great as these muscle men are. I understand also that many aren't just training to be a competitive bodybuilders, but they do want to tighten up their physique and achieve that coveted athletic look that you see on the cover of "Women's Fitness Magazine's".

Well,regardless of what kind of athletic look you may be after, this book will help you to achieve the type of physique your looking for. Building muscle for women takes hard work, nothing comes easy. But we will show you how with the correct exercises , dietary modifications, and nutritional supplements how to achieve that perfect looking type of body that so many women envy.

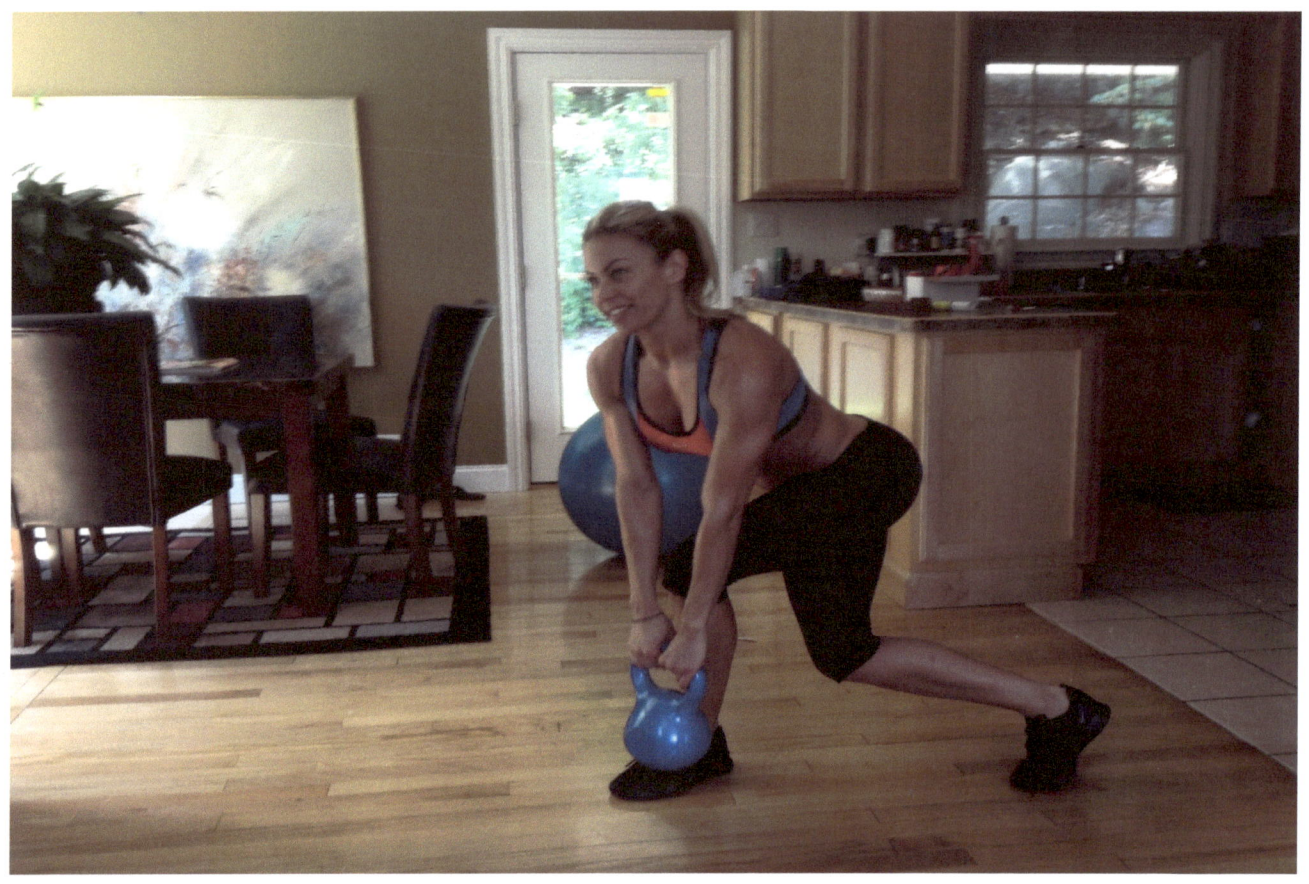

Chapter 1
Getting Real About Women & Muscle Gain

I'm not talking about the women that have muscles looking like male bodybuilders, these women obviously are on synthetic steroids, and male testosterone. You have to realize that women have a fraction of testosterone than what male bodybuilders do, but that's not to say that they can't build a muscular body with a simple dietary change in foods and supplements.

With the proper nutritional guidance and training routine, they can have a look that would be the envy of many women. Studies show that men and women do not need to train differently. So if your a women, and want to train and have a muscular body or just want to tighten up, then your going to have to train with weights.

Men and women do not need to train differently to see results , nor should they eat differently than men do either, but there are some modifications that are different when it comes to nutritional supplementation. Men and women's metabolism are very similar, except that women burn a greater ratio of fat to carb's than men do. This is one one the reasons why women do well on low carb diets.

Women need fewer calories than men because they have more muscle mass to fat than men, and that is the main thing that needs to be adjusted. So when it comes to diet for a women's training ,the amount of protein, carbs, and fat will be dictated by the amount of calories she eats. If you are a women trying to gain lean muscle mass, you will then need to consume adequate amounts of protein and essential fatty acids in your diet.

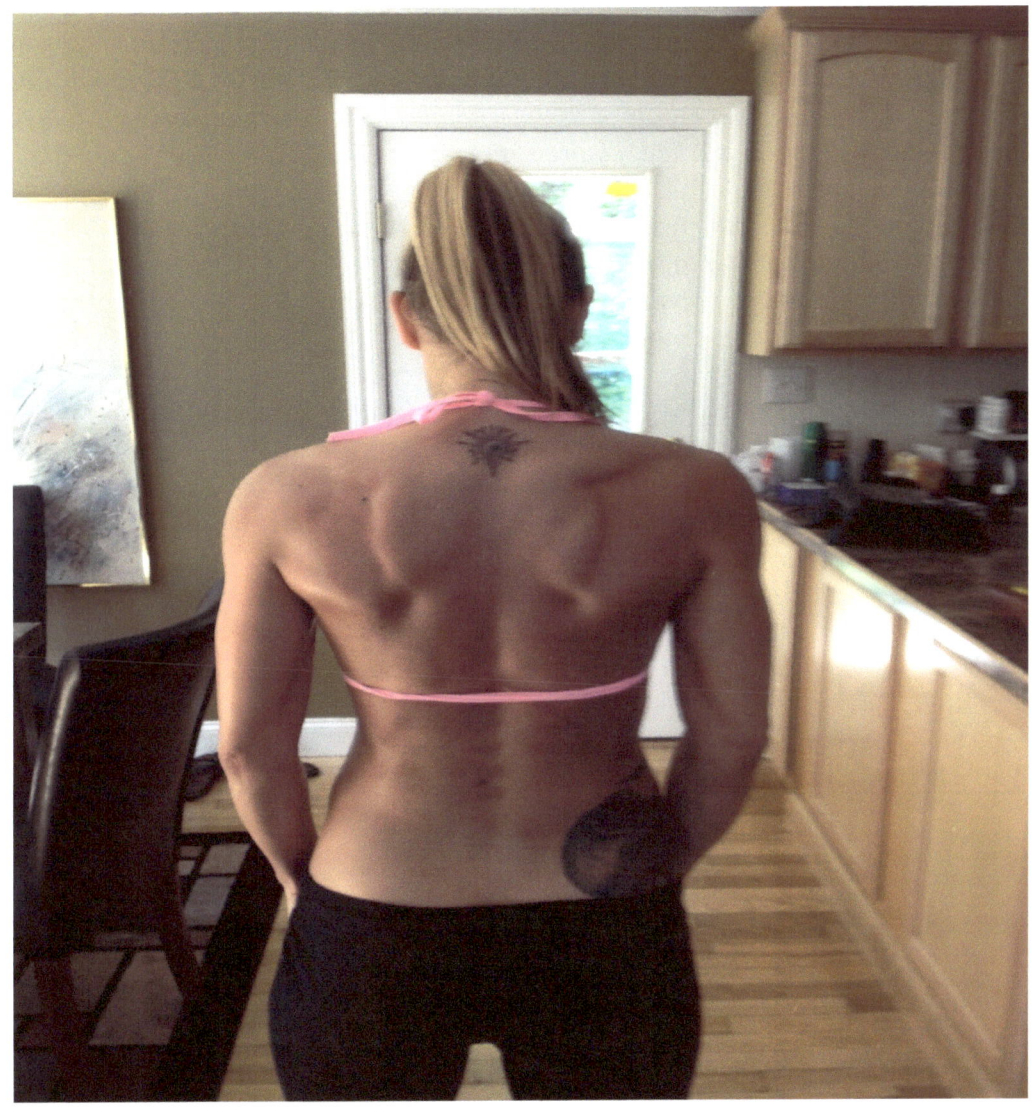

Chapter 2
Workout Diet & Nutrition For Women

Let's face it,when it comes to building a good looking muscular body, 90% of the results will depend on nutrition and diet. If you do not eat properly, you won't build the body that you want. Many men and women who training for that athletic look spend most of their time designing a workout routine and types of exercise that their going to employ.

They focus most of their attention on fancy split routines, but have no clue on how much protein, calories, or carb's they are eating per day. To build muscle you need to focus more so on your dietary needs than training, that comes secondary. Because when you eat right and take the necessary supplements , you will definitely gain the muscle so desired.

A muscle building diet plan is different than just eating healthy, it has specific requirements that must be met if you are going to succeed in achieving your fitness goal.

<u>Here are the specific breakdown of required foods</u>:

⚔ **Proteins** – *this is a must in monitoring your protein needs as protein intake is very important in feeding the muscles. You have to remember that muscle tissue is on a constant turn over rate when doing resistance type of training, from building lean muscle to tissue repair and recovery. To maximize this growth and repair of tissue you must keep your body in a positive nitrogen retention balance. Protein is a key requirement.*

⚔ **Carbohydrates** – *Carb's play two vital roles in your diet, one is maximizing your energy levels required for training and two to spike your insulin levels to drive nutrients into your blood stream. Insulin is the most anabolic hormone the produces, and if managed correctly it can help you maximize your growth potential.*

⚔ **Essential Healthy Fatty Acids** – *The body requires healthy fats for a number of reasons, hormonal balance, brain metabolism, and a healthy cardiovascular system. Under eating these healthy fatty acids can compromise slow recovery from training sessions, sleeping ability, cardiovascular function and the likely hood of over training.*

⚔ **Calories** – *Under eating your calories can be one of the reasons that your not making any gains. You must eat a substantial amount of calories on a daily basis to allow your body to make muscle.*

Choosing The Right Amount of Protein:

Although there are many protein ratio per pound of body weight recommendations, we will stick with something a little more in the muscle building realm of things so as not to confuse things. Instead of relying on these ratio's per pound of body weight, it is much more easier if we stick to this guide line.

Try and eat 30 to 40 grams of protein every 3 hours.

By using this as a guide line, you will be consuming about 150 to a little 200 grams of protein on a daily basis. In general 180 grams to 220 grams would be considered sufficient for most natural weight lifters.

Choosing The Right Amount Of Fatty Acid Intake

Your essential fat intake should basically compromise 20% to 30% of your daily caloric intake. Fat contains 9 calories per gram, compared to protein and carbohydrates which contain 4 calories per gram which makes fat calories more dense. *If you do need to add more calories , remember to just add more essential fats to your die*t.

Choosing Your Carbohydrate Intake

Carbohydrates are the preferred form of energy your muscles require and are stored in the in the body in limited amounts as "glycogen" in muscles and in the liver. When exercising the body uses all of its glycogen, and if you can not maintain your exercise intensity, then your glycogen levels are depleted.

The following chart will help you determine your carbohydrate intake based on your body weight. In general athletes require about 3.1 to 4.5 grams of carbs per day per pound of body weight. Putting it in a more perspective way , non-athletes require 1.8 to 2.3 grams of carbs per pound of body weight.

Carbohydrate Needs For Athletes

Training Level	Grams of Carbohydrate per pound per day
1 hour of training	2.7 to 3.1 grams
2 hours of training	3.6 grams
3 hours of training	5 grams
4 hours of training	5.5 to 5.9 grams

Choosing Health Foods That Add Calories Fast

If you are having a difficult time in choosing health foods to add calories to your diet,the following list of foods below are calorie dense.

- *Wheat Pasta*
- *Whole Grain Wheat Cereals*
- *Almonds and Nuts*
- *Natural Peanut Butter & Almond Butter*
- *Avocado's*
- *Banana's*
- *Beef*
- *Butter,Natural*
- *Olive Oil*
- *Natural Unfiltered Pure Honey*
- *Dark Chocolate*
- *Cheese*
- *Whole Milk*

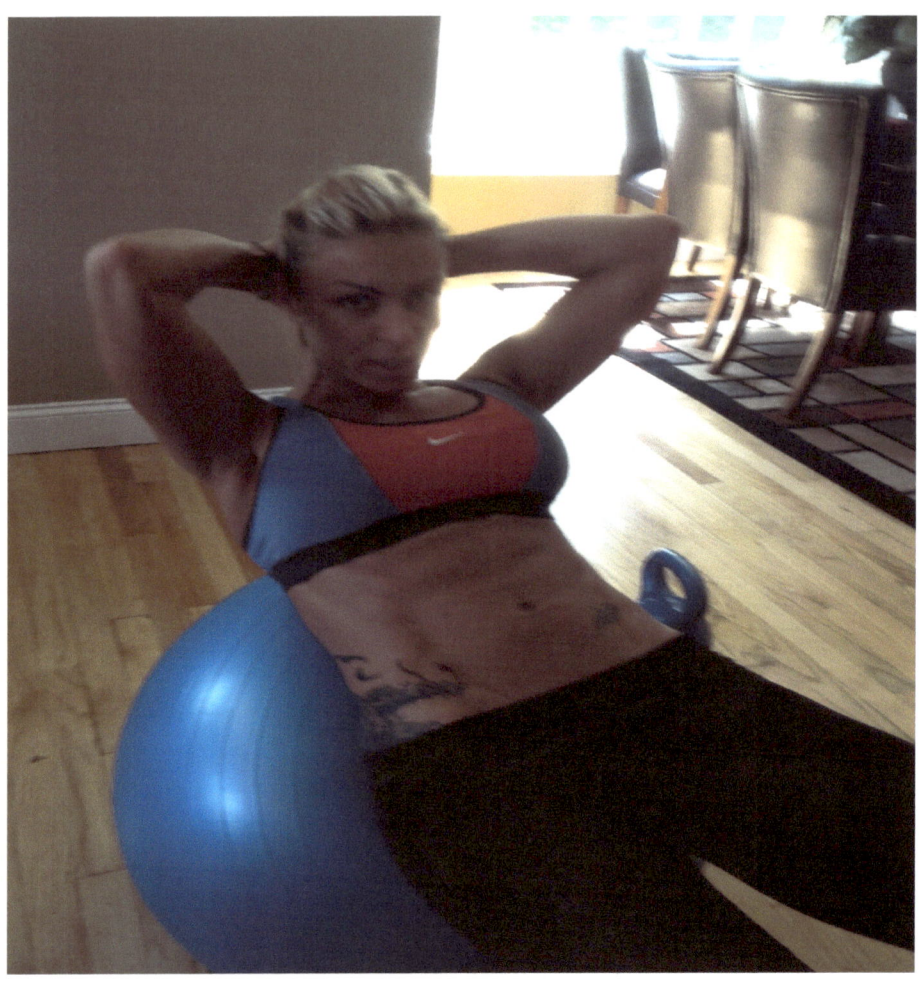

Chapter 3
How To Plan Your Bodybuilding Meals

By combining the proper foods, you could create an anabolic effect. 90% of of the battle in bodybuilding pertains to dietary nutrition. We are after all what we eat. I'm not trying to say that you will get the same effects as steroid user's, but you will definitely be close.

However your results and effort will far surpass anything that you are currently experiencing now, and I promise you that! In a moment or so you will be introduced in a nutritional strategy that will revolutionize your muscle fitness life. You will make gains in lean muscularity and with no addition of body fat, and yes ! You can build muscle and lose body fat at the same time.

This nutritional strategy works and was tried out by myself and the cover model that is on the cover of this book , as well as many others that followed the methods in this book. If you implement this information and process it wisely, you will make gains like never before.
This method does take planning on your part and if you stay committed it will be well worth it for you.

This nutritional strategy will maximize your natural anabolic hormones – estrogen, testosterone,GH,and insulin.
How To Structure Your Meal Plans

The easiest way to approach your daily eating plan is to structure everything around, breakfast,lunch,and dinner. In between meals , or later you can add healthy snacks. These snacks will allow you to add the additional protein and nutrients that you'll need to help you recover and build lean muscle growth.

<u>Note</u>: *In between snacks are those that are extremely thin and just starting out with the program.*

<u>**Your Calculations:**</u>

Calories – 15 calories per pound/body weight
Protein – 1 to 1.5 grams per pound/body weight
Carbs – 1.4 grams per pound/body weight

There are going to be several differences between the nutritional plan for non-workouts and on workout days. Being that there will be no additional energy expenditures on non-workout days, the pre-workout and post workout meals are combined into one meal. It is mostly carbohydrates that are reduced in order to suit the reduced energy needs of the body on the non-workout days.

However even on non-workout days protein intake still remains to be high in order to focus on maximizing muscle growth. On non-workout days fat consumption should also remain to be high as well, since experience has shown that that people with low body fat levels recover better and faster if the fat intake comprises at least one third of their daily caloric intake, and for this reason 120 grams of fat should be consumed on non-workout days , which equals out to 1100 calories.

It is also best to use a various combination of fast and slow protein sources like lean ground beef, medium fat cheese,and whole organic eggs should be consumed for this purpose shortly before going to bed. Rapid muscle growth can only occur if you if you allow for a steady supply of high quality nutrients.

In regards to supplementation, you would want to take 5 to 10 grams of powdered **<u>Colostrum</u>** two times a day to allow for maximum anabolic growth. **<u>Colostrum</u>** is becoming very popular with athletes in the know of this amazing supplement that is rich in natural growth factors like IgF-1,amino acids,vitamins,minerals,immuno-globulins, and anti-bodies.

We also would like to add **<u>Vitargo-CGL by Nutrex</u>**, one serving per day to further speed up the recovery process and to expand muscle cell volume via creating and glycogen induced super hydration. It is best to consume Vitargo-CGL immediately upon rising in the morning on non-workout days. Knowing that insulin sensitivity is also at its peak.

<u>*Note: Try and drink at least one gallon of water per day.*</u>

<u>**Example Combination of Meal Planning :**</u>

In general Pick Foods That Build muscle With High Quality Nutrients From Each Food Group.

<u>**Sample Meal Plans:**</u>

<u>**Meal -1**</u>

Vegetable omlet (3 egg whites,1 whole egg, 1 cup veg's) you could also add some lean beef or chicken breast.

Meal -2

One cup yogurt or protein shake.

Meal – 3

6 oz. Chicken breast or turkey (white meat)
small raw vegetable salad
1 bagel

Meal – 4

1 piece fruit
3-4 oz chicken breast or turkey (white meat)

Meal – 5

6 oz. Of fish -salmon
1 cup grilled veggies
1 cup brown rice

Sample Meal Plan #2

Meal – 1

3 packs of instant oatmeal
1 banana
1 cup yougurt
*1 cup cottage chees*e

Meal -2

Protein shake
1 large baked potato

Meal – 3

8 oz chicken breast
2 cups pasta
1 apple
1 cup yogurt

Meal -4

1 cup Tuna
1-2 cups broccoli

Meal – 5

Protei shake
1 cup brown rice

Meal – 6

8 oz broiled fish salmon
1 cup veggies
2 cups brown rice

Sample Meal Plan -#3

Meal -1

3 Egg whites,` whole egg, 1 cup chopped onions/green pepper/red pepper
1 cup cottage cheese
1 cup blue berries

Meal – 2

Protein shake
1 cup raw veggies

Meal – 3

Salmon burger on whole wheat bread,1 egg white,cooked onions
1 large potato
1 garden salad

Meal – 4

Protein shake
1 cup yogurt

Meal – 5

8 oz chicken breast cut in chunks ,fried in olive oil seasoned with garlic,peppers,onions
2 cups pasta
1 cup broccoli

Meal – 6

Protein shake
1 cup melon
1 cup yougurt

There is no need to carefully measure for exact portions suggested ! Just eyeball your portions and consider the chart below:

1 oz meat = match book size
3 oz meat = deck of cards
8 oz meat =thin paper back book
3 oz fish =check book
1 oz of cheese =four dice
1 cup pasta = tennis ball

Nutrition plays a very lasrge part in bodybuilding and growth and remember that bodybuilding diets are constantly changing due to the increase in your muscle mass, for example if you put on more muscle mass you have to eat more,if lose muscle you need to eat less.

So how do we keep an eye on whats happening to our body? Well the first rule is to monitor your eight and progress to see if your goal to put muscle on is causing an increase in body weight and muscle. The second way is to check whether muscle or fat is going up by the means of using a body fat caliper. By using a body fat caliper, is a good way to determine every two weeks or so if you need to eat more or need to eat less. Body fat calipers show fat percentages with in the body and is a good indicator regarding your progress.

The above meal plans are just examples of types meals you should be employing to give you an idea of what types of foods you should be eating. You can mix this around to suit your needs or goals , but basically this should do the trick.

Conclusion In Summary

Important points to Remember.....**If your not gaining weight** – eat twice the amount of carb's and 1.5 times as much protein at two of your meals during the course of the day.

If you are gaining weight, but its just as much muscle as fat then – Eliminate your carb intake at your last two meals of the day,including your post workout- meal.

If you did fine at first , but now your body fat has increased – then you must have your carb's at your last two meals, if your body fat falls off in two weeks, then increase your carb's.

If your gaining muscle and losing fat – well, then your on the right track ,and keep it up !

Remember To Rest – on your off days,remember to relax and give your body ample amount of rest to recover for your next training session.Try and keep intense training sessions down to 2 – 3 days a week.

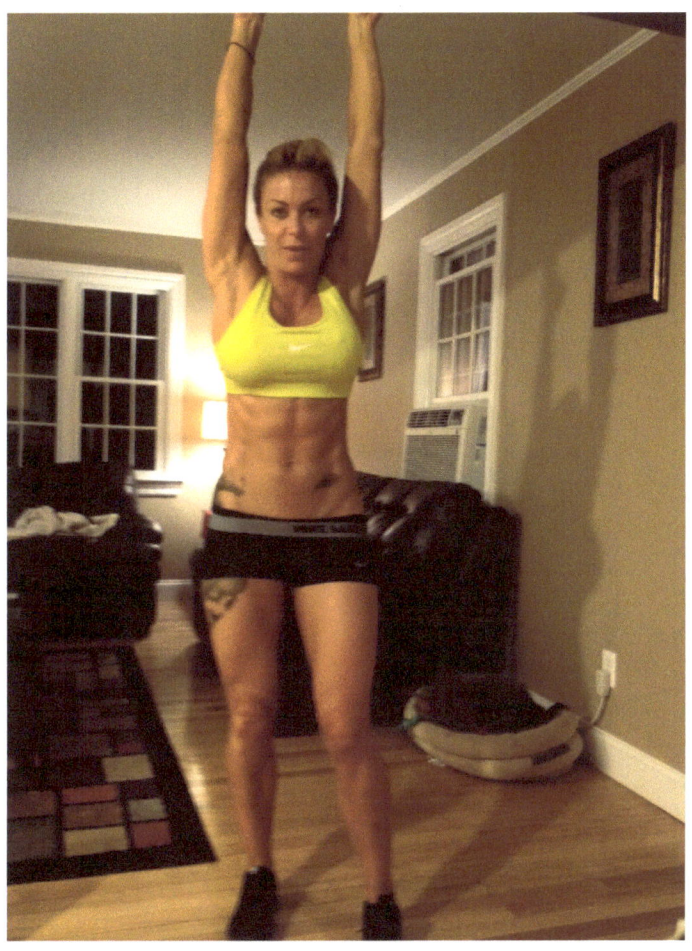

Chapter 4
How to Access Leaner Body Fat Percentages in Female Athletes

In general women have a higher percentage of body fat than men do , mainly because their reproductive hormones require more body fat. Their general body fat percentage is between 15% and 25% , and in the mens it fall between 10% to 20% . Optimal body fat levels for women athletes are 10% to 20% and 5% to 12% for men athletes.

<u>**Body Fat Percentage in Athletes and Non-athletes**</u>

<u>Women</u>		<u>Men</u>
Athlete	**10 – 20%**	**15 – 20%**
Normal	**15-20%**	**10 – 20%**
Overweight	**25 – 29%**	**20 - 24%**
Obese	**over 30%**	**over 25%**

As a women you can also have too little body fat as well, this is not a healthy matter as having body fat levels of less than 12% can compromise hormonal function in which menstruation can be interrupted and increase the risk of osteoporosis. Body fat levels of 10% in women and 4% in men may be an indication of an eating disorder. Just remember that your body some essential fats considered to be about 10 to 4 to 10% in men and 10% to 12% minimum for women to help with the manufacture of hormones,vitamins,minerals,and amino acids.

The Ultimate Female Training Guide:Proven Methods To Get Lean Muscle

Its always been the primary concern for women when they begin a weight training program that they do not want to get too big and bulky !   Well I'm here to tell you that you won't.

It is the hormone testosterone that is responsible for large increases in muscle mass when lifting weights. But a womens testosterone levels are only a fraction of what a man's level puts out. A normal blood level of testosterone for a man is 200-1200ng/dl while a womens level falls under 15-70ng/dl , and as you can see a man's level is much higher.

When it comes down to training, studies have shown that men and women need not training differently. If you are a women and you want to develop your shape and improve your curves , you then must lift with heavy weights and challenge yourself in a progressive way that will stimulate lean muscle growth.

Here is an overview of the rep ranges that will help you in determining an ideal balance of rep schemes to your weight training needs.

Strength – 1 to 5 reps

Hypertrophy – 6 to 12 reps

Endurance – 12 reps and up.

This gives you an idea of the weight that you'll need in order to grow. This is just a superficial idea of what most people grow muscle on. Six to 12 reps seems to be the normal rep range completing 6 reps but not more than 12. It can not stressed enough that you use strict form in all your exercise movements.

<u>**Warm – Ups**</u>

You should always warm up properly before beginning your training session. One to three sets is usually sufficient enough to get your circulation to your muscles going to avoid any injury to your body.

<u>**Rest Peroids In Between Sets**</u>

It is generally recommended to give your muscles 60 to 120 seconds of rest in between sets. The whole point is when training you would want to up the tempo and keep a good blood flow to the the muscle group your training, you want to get in and get out ,and trying to accomplish in 45 minutes to no more than one hour in the gym.

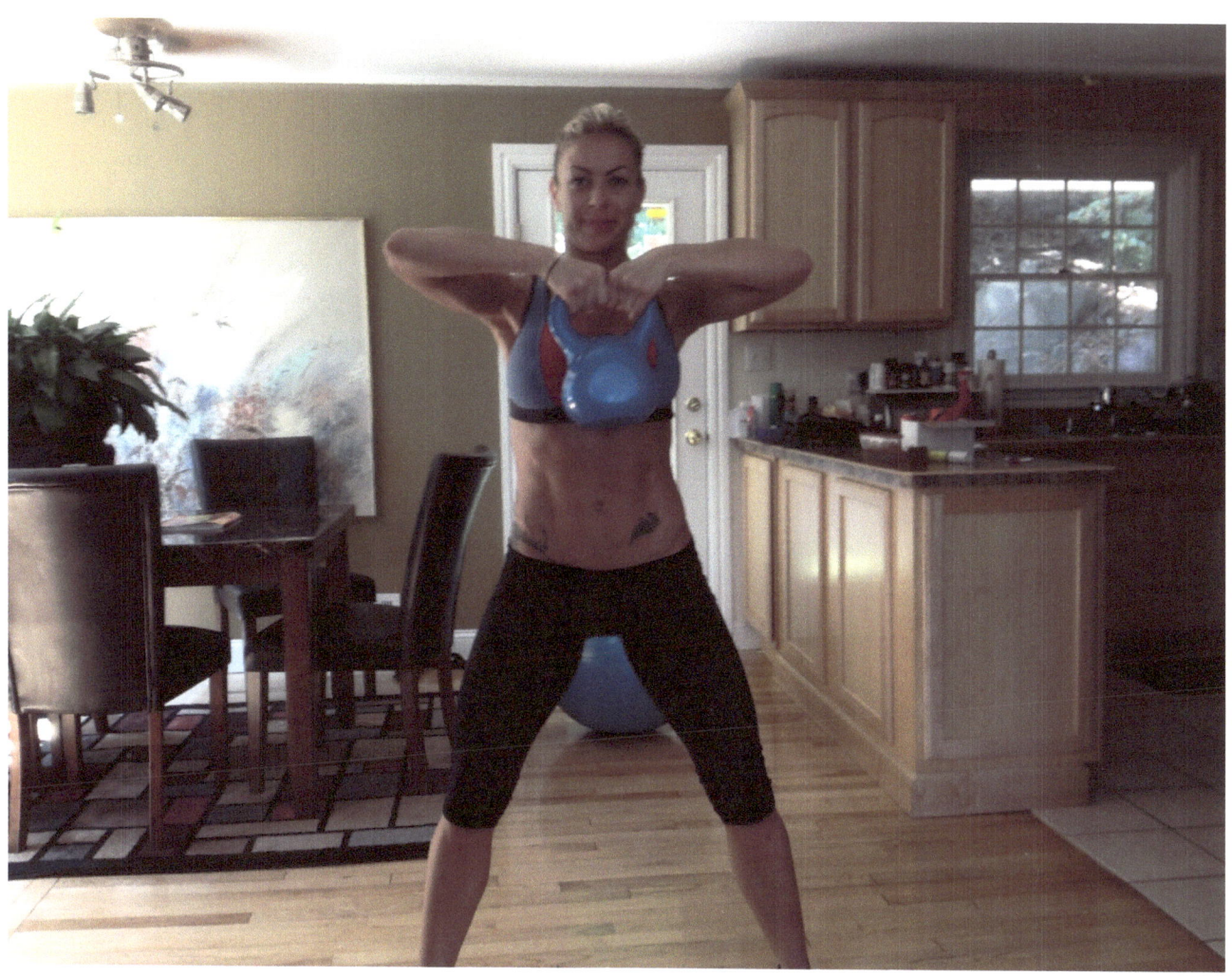

Chapter 5
Working The Trouble Area's of The Body

Almost everyone has certain trouble areas of the body that they would like to work on and improve. These are areas where most of the body fat accumulates and is stored. In most women these are the difficult areas that we are going to show you how to eliminate these unwanted and trouble fatty deposits like the thighs,glutes (butt), love handles, and in some women the tricep area in the back of the arm that when you wave hello or good buy , it waves back to you !

The most important thing to remember is after dieting to lose weight and tone up these trouble spots the last thing that you would want to do is gain back this excess fat. So if you don't learn to keep your diet clean and know what to eat to stay lean and keep what you earned you'll wind up gaining the fat back. Diet is more than half the battle in any exercise program. Exercises are merely tools that we employ to tone up and build our body to the desired level that we choose.

The Most Effective Exercises For Those Trouble Area's

In general these are the most effective and productive exercises that can be a potent formula that you can use over and over again to tone up or build up into a physique that will be admire by many of your peers.

- ⅄ **The following 7 exercises are arguably the best for fast results.**

- ⅄ <u>**Barbell Squats**</u> – **This is the king of all overall body exercise's that affects your thighs,and overall body strength. Squats tax the whole body in general and should be performed as strict as possible with buttocks touching the ankles on the way down. Inhaling and exhaling as you go up and down. Sets should be 2-3 and rep range from 6 to 12 pyramiding up to 12 with the last set. Do not count your warm up as your first set,but make sure you warm up thoroughly before you begin your first set.**

- ⅄ <u>**Deadlifts**</u> – **This exercise is second only to squats in terms of building and toning overall body development. It is also important to wear a weightlifting belt when performing this particular exercise in avoiding back injury. When done correctly this movement gets results fast ! Warm-up are also important, so make sure you warm up before beginning this movement. Sets and rep range are the same as squats.**

- ⅄ <u>**Dips**</u> – **This exercise is done on a parallel bar using your own bodyweight. As you progress you can also add weight with a make shift strap chain that goes around your waist with the added weight secured in the middle. One of the great upper body exercises thats actually a favorite of mine. Improvements are seen within a week or so when done properly. Sets are 2-to 3 with reps done in a pyramid fashion,6 to 12 .**

- ⅄ <u>**Barbell Bench Press**</u> – **A great upper body developer that targets most of your upper body muscles with the pectorals being the main focus here, but also affecting the shoulders,and triceps. There are also other variations of this exercise that you can do, like flat,incline,or decline which shifts the focus on different area's of the upper body. Sets should be 2-3 and reps 6 to 12.**

- ⅄ <u>**Pull-Ups**</u> – **This is an excellent exercise for building and shaping the upper back muscles, also affecting the biceps. This exercise is done using your bodyweight ,and as you progress you can also add more weight in the same manner as was spoken with the dips. 2 to 3 sets should be enough , with reps being 6 to 12.**

- ⅄ <u>**Overhead Military Barbell or Dumbell Press**</u> - **This exercise can be done seated on a bench or standing. Overhead press's are another solid choice for complete shoulder development. Sets and reps are the same as above.**

- ⅄ <u>**Barbell Rowing or Dumbell Rowing**</u> – **Both variations are very effective in building and shaping your complete back development along with your biceps. Sets and reps are the same as above.**

There is no need to add to this routine as it is sufficient enough in producing the results that you striving for. You can always up the intensity as you further progress into the weeks. Your body will become stronger and your endurance will increase, so by raising the intensity level you will realize that you will complete the program at a much quicker pace.

After 6 to 8 weeks you an split the variations of exercises that can be done with a barbell or dumbell.

Example -

Barbell Bench Press / Dumbell Bench Press
Barbell Rowing /Dumbell Rowing (done with one arm at a time)
Barbell Military Press / Dumbell Press

Preliminary Warm-ups Before Beginning Your training Sessions

Know that the process of warming up actually involves three important phases.

Stretching – Do several minutes of full body stretching that are specific to your training sessions.
Cardio – 5 to 10 minutes of a non-taxing cardio session.

Prepare your body and mind for your training session by focusing on your specific exercises at hand. All movements should be done at a specific pace never resting more than your required time limit,60 to 120 seconds.

Training For Longevity and Keeping Fit

Aging, a normal process that is part of life as we get past the age of 50, we lose certain functions, muscle tone,strength,and flexibility. But we can do something to prolong this dilemma. By manipulating certain lifestyle factors like exercise,a good dietary food plan and supplements to support our nutritional needs we can keep an active lifestyle and set the aging clock back by 10 years or so. Just look at the great exercise pioneers like Jack Lalanne that exercised well into his 90's and lived to the fruitful age of 96.The father of fitness always advocated how important it was to employ a sound exercise program supplemented with a good nutritional diet was the key ! As they say, use it or lose it !

The Pillars of Wellness and Fitness

Doing both aerobic exercises and strength training will enhance your muscular strength and improve your cardiovascular system by bringing blood flow to your heart,muscles, and lungs.
Healthy Eating Plan is especially important as we aging our later years,so its important to include fresh fruits,vegetables,whole grains and high quality proteins. Also eliminating junk foods,processed foods, preservatives, nitrates,and all these artificial sweeteners. America today has become a lazy nation always looking for something that comes in a pill form to achieve what we desire. That is not the way, for its been proven for many years now that studies do show that we can extend our youth well into our senior years.

For longevity purposes ,exercises build muscle and lean body mass. It is this loss of body mass that leads to an overall decline in aging and in the quality of life. Exercise is the single most important factor in the aspect of us living a healthy and active life. When it comes to anti-aging exercising, resistance training does several things to the body that are critical to our well being, first it builds muscle and burns fat.

Its also an important factor in preventing muscle wasting syndrome and osteoporosis. Aerobic training or cardiovascular training plays a different role in promoting longevity which is to improve and maintain the hearts ability to supply oxygen to the body and vital organs. There are certain recommendations for cardiovascular training that an individual needs to get their heart rate up to 80%

and keep it there for a maximum time of 15 to 20 minutes three times a week. This can be incorporated into your training session in which I would recommend on the off days of your workouts.

Many experts believe that strength training is the key to prevent age related decline and disabilities. If you don't exercise as you age you loose muscle mass and it could have all kinds of implications such as heart disease,type 2 diabetes and other chronic illness's. The important thing to remember is that one is never to old to start exercising. The human body has an amazing ability to respond to exercise no matter what age. In studies done with senior citizens in their 80's or older showed that they gained strength just as rapidly as a younger person did.

<u>Health experts all agree that resistance training rejuvenates your health in the following ways-</u>

- ⚔ Prevents muscle wasting syndrome.
- ⚔ Benefits your cardiovascular system.
- ⚔ Strengthens your bones.
- ⚔ Improves flexibility.
- ⚔ Prevents disease and illness.
- ⚔ Prevents and fights diabetes.

With average life expectancy at about 75 to 77 years old , hat the quality of our life is just as important as the amount of candles on our cake. Now you know its possible to increase the quality of your lifestyle and improve every aspect of your well being,your muscles,your athletic look,healing time, and regain your youth.

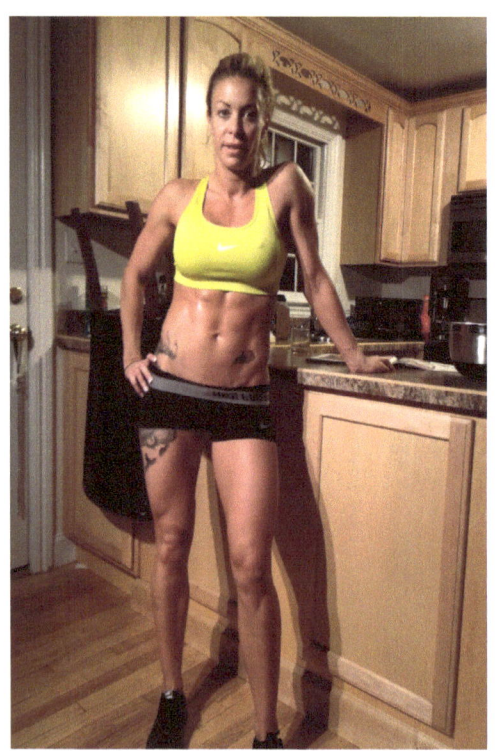

Chapter 6
Restoring Youth Through Exercise, Diet and Nutritional Supplements

Studies have have shown that the single most important factor in long lived people around the world is the retention of muscle mass. With the right combination of exercises such as strength training ,which research shows releases natural growth hormone, a protein hormone with its certain amino acid sequence that is highly beneficial in restoring the anti-aging clock back coercing the rejuvenation of a healthy body.

Beneficial Exercises & Proven Ways that Stimulate Gh-Release

Squats – offers a high volume form of resistance that supports the release of GH.

Rowing- whether its with a machine or barbells and dumbells also triggers a gh response right from the pituitary gland. Incorporate high repetitions.

Cycling – during intense cycling the lactic acid build-up that is generated -(the burning effect) that is often felt, raises the bar called "lactic acid threshold" of intensity extends gh-release.

Deadlifts – a good overall body developer that helps with a surge of gh-release that will strengthen overall body mass quickly.

Pull-Ups – this gh release list would not be complete with this great overall upper body developer. Considered the mother of all upper body exercises.

Sleep -going to bed on an empty stomach with carbohydrates, carb's help the body to produce insulin, and insulin is a gh agnostic helping the body store fat. Your body will only produce one at a time, insulin or gh.

Training –doing short high intensity workouts at least two times a week. Squats, deadlifts, and rowing.

Getting Enough Sleep –a sound deep sleep is a great gh-releaser which is produced within the first hour or so. Naps also help !

Eating -eating high protein foods with ample amino acid's which are precursor's to gh production.

List of Amino Acids That Support GH-Release

⚓ **Glutamine** – 2,000 mgs.,Research showed that 2 grams of glutamine had a stimulating affect on Gh production. Most athletes that are over trained were found to be depleted in glutamine.

⚓ **Arginine** -2 to 4 grams, currently a hot item in many gh formula's. Also required in the production of GH. Another important factor is arginine's ability to boost nitric oxide levels in the body. Thus making arginine a potential aid in the treatment of cardiovascular function and support.

⚓ **Ornithinine** -2 to 4 grams.,Often combined with arginine in a 2:1 ratio as a potent combination in the manufacture of growth hormone.

- **Lysine** -2 grams,considered an essential amino acid thats required for growth and bone development. It also helps to regulate the pineal gland and ovaries.

- **Gaba** - 500mgs to 1,000mgs, an amino acid inhibitory neurotransmitter gamma aminobutryic acid has been shown to raise serum growth hormone level concentrations in test subjects. Gaba has a calming effect similar to the popular anti-anxiety drug valium.

- **L-Dopa** (mucuna prureins) 60% extract or higher - 100 to 200 mgs two times a day. L-Dopa , a powerful neurotransmitter precursor to dopamine an essential componet of the functioning of the brain. L-Dopa contains natural secretagogues that help in the manufacture of growth hormone. Used extensively in gh releasing formula's as a main ingredient.

- **Glycine** -4 grams,a non-essential amino acid which early research showed its ability to increase strength in athletes. More recent studies also revealed its ability in raising plasma growth hormone levels in humans.

All amino acids should always be taken on an empty stomach before bed or one hour before training sessions.

Natural Co-factors & Nutrients That Stimulate GH-Release

DMAE – helps generate acetylcholine in the brain which helps with the production of raising growth hormone levels.

Vitamin – C - required for the synthesis of amino acids in the manufacture of gh production.

DHEA – a slight androgenic hormone produced by the adrenal glands of males and females that declines with age. Studies on animals does show that DHEA promotes longer life span by helping the body stimulate gh release by means of regulating insulin levels.

Melatonin – has been well publicized and highly lauded as a natural sleep aid and longevity supplement. A powerful anti-oxidant as well and potent gh-releaser in its own right. 1 to 3 mgs has been shown to raise GH levels by 157%. Natural melatonin levels decline with age and that would explain why some older individuals have insomnia. Adding melatonin to your personal supplement protocol can benefit you in leading a healthy and productive lifestyle.

Niacin - (B3) - a potent vasodilator ,500mgs of niacin has been known to stimulate gh-release and helps to prevent or reverse cardiovascular disorder by helping to lower cholesterol levels in the body. You will find niacin in many gh-enhancer formula's on the market today. Please note that niacin will cause a flushing effect, sort of like a hot flash which is harmless and normally subsides after 15 minutes or so. It normally goes away when taken on a regular basis.

Vitamin B6 - needed for amino acid synthesis in the conversion of GH. Also used as a cofactor in many GH formula's as well.

Ornithine Alpha-Ketoglutarate (OKG) – the amino acids ornithine and glutamine are combined to form ornithine alpha-ketoglutarate (OKG). OKG enhances the body's release of growth hormone and insulin and increases arginine and glutamine levels in the muscle tissue. A good anti-catabolic ,OKG also helps prevent the breakdown of muscle tissue.

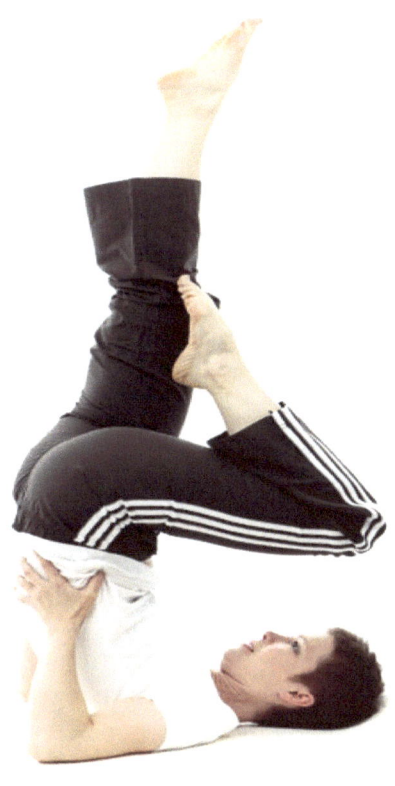

Chapter 7
Popular Natural GH-Releasing Formulas

Deer Antler Velvet - considered the most purest and potent form of Deer Antler Velvet product out in the market today. This product is taking the fitness world over because of its natural growth hormone and IgF-1 effects on the human body. Made very popular with the players of the National Football League and Major League Baseball .The effects are extraordinary and rejuvenating. A must try product that you will feel and notice the effects within two to three days of use. Can be purchased on line by Nutronic's Labs.com. Nutronic's sells 8 different formula's and the most potent of them all is "IgF-1+ . Deer Antler Velvet is now a recognized source of an important insulin-growth-factors (IgF-1) and IgF-2,isolated after the velvet is scraped off the antlers, and then dried and sprayed. Deer Antler Velvet has been used in traditional Chinese Medicine for centuries, because it works !
Deer Antler Velvet which also first became available in the United States just a dozen years ago , that guarantees its users that over 90% of them will receive and experience atleast 7 of the 25 typical benefits within the first month of use.

IgF-1+ by "Now Sports" - also an excellent product that is actually manufactured by nutronic's labs. Just a weaker version but still very effective and gets results !

Powerful -by USP Labs - a very potent extract of mucuna prureins (L-Dopa) that more than doubles the release of GH. Powerful has also been the subject on multiple studies on its growth hormone releasing effect. An excellent product to use both in and out of the gym.

Secretropin – this product was developed by Dr.Gordon based on 9 years of clinical research on natural GH releasers. The formula is based on two amino acids ,arginine and ornithine. His findings based on his product were increased levels of IgF-1 and IgFBP-3, two important markers of growth hormone production. What was impressive in the study , was an average increase in IgF-1 of 50 to 200% that was documented in 92 percent of the participants that took his product. See www.raisemygh.com for further information.

Royal Jelly – excellent product, full of nutritional compounds and growth factors. Royal Jelly given to the queen bee as a food source by the worker bee's. A rich source of B-vitamins,amino acids,fatty acids, trace minerals,and enzymes. Royal Jelly can not be duplicated in the laboratory and can only be made by nature. Royal Jelly also has the potential to rejuvenate your pituitary gland to produce more GH. Used by many cultures throughout the world for its medicinal value and healing affects, Royal Jelly can have a very positive and beneficial affect on your health and rejuvenation.

When buying Royal Jelly, make sure it was kept cold as it is very temperature sensitive. It can be purchased from amazon.com or your local natural health food store.

Note: Conclusion

Hopefully by now you have some kind of idea of solid understanding of how nutritional supplements can have an affect on our biological function on growth hormone and muscle cell growth. Knowing now that secretion of GH declines as we age , we can improve and slow down the effects of aging as it relates to muscle and fitness. I have given you the top proven GH releasing supplements out there that work best for providing you of which ones to use and to make them part of your everyday nutritional regimen.

To simplify things a bit easier for you, I would start on the basic already made formula that are listed the popular GH releasing formula's, and judge for yourself by how you feel, and from results that you get.

Dietary Foods That Help Increase Hormonal Health

By combing proper nutrition with appropriate exercise's and the necessary supplements
you then have the tools to create a vibrant healthy lifestyle that will create a fully lived,long and healthy life.

The biggest problems we face today as Americans is obesity. More than half of us are over our ideal weight and more than one-third are obese enough to significantly raise their risk's of disease and a premature death. Nutrition and eating correctly are one of the greatest tools we have against leading a healthy lifestyle and eliminating disease.A rcent study showed that eating daily servings of fruits and vegetables, along with three servings of healthy fatty acids lowers your risk of getting heart disease,cancer, and can be as effective as medication in lowering high blood pressure and reducing or eliminate your chance's of getting a stroke.

In this chapter we will look into the health foods that help regulate and manufacture hormonal function in the body, and some of which are considered super foods ! Foods to consider in, as it was once said by the Father of Medicine "Hippocrates" an ancient Greek physician that was considered on of the most outstanding figures in the history of medicine , that stated "Let Thy Food Be Thy Medicine" is fact that we lose sight of .

As a natural holistic health practitioner these words do figure so true! For I've seen what natural healthfoods can do, because we are what we eat ! And disease does manifest in the stomach first, if you eat incorrectly, you don't function in a healthy state. I hope that I have shed some light on the importance of eating healthy to remain disease free. So lets begin in starting with the top foods that will super charge your body like you never thought possible till you read here in this book.

Top Super Foods To Super Charge Your Health

Overview: Super foods are foods that have an incredible array of health benefits that go well beyond their nutritional value in the human body.

Goji Berries – Goji Berries are the only food that will help you produce more natural growth hormone directly . Considered one of the most potent super foods and anti-aging tonics in the world. Just by eating a handful of these nutritious berries on a daily basis, you will be providing your body with the necessary nutrients and potent anti-oxidants to enhance your GH levels,immune system,and your longevity. Goji berries can be consumed in a smoothie type of shake,eaten plain, or made in a tea to extract the medicinal qualities. This is one food that should be made an everyday snack, trust me you will thank me later !

Noni Juice – Also known as (morinda citrifolia) Noni juice has always been a hot topic among health professionals for its outstanding health producing effects, with its strong healing affect and potential still remaining a secret. Considered a Polynesian fruit that has been used there as a powerful medicine and health tonic. Noni juice supposedly cures every disease under the sun. Still, scientists today are corroborating newer findings
about noni with clinical studies and in depth research.
Noni Juce is know to be rich in phytochemicals that can help in the treatment and prevention of many diseases known today. The applications that noni can have affect on is just too many to get into detail, but to just name a few noni can improve your moods and sleep,blood circulation,act as a powerful anti-inflammatory,powerful pain reliever,
improve skin tone and health,immuno-stimulant,anti-viral,ant-bacterial,anti-fungal,and most the natives in Polynesia just consume it as an anti-aging factor.But you name it and noni seems to cure it !
When purchasing noni juice,make sure that your noni juice is pure, certified and concentrated. Also first time users of noni juice will have an affect of a natural elimination of bodily impurites and toxins as it detoxifies the body, so you may notice some pimples,boils, or gas and diarrhea. Nothing to be alarmed about !

Maca - Organic Maca powder that comes from raw maca. This is a natural adaptogenic root known for its dynamic effect on regulating the body's hormones. Loaded with beneficial nutrients and highly prized in Peru and South America, Maca will benefit your health in a miraculous way. Sometimes prepared and eaten as a root vegetable for its nutritional and medicinal assests, maca will regulate everything to do with hormonal function.

Chlorella (CGF) - A therapeutic green algae that has been in existence for almost 2 billion years, that grows narurally in lakes and ponds. Chlorella also has the ability to quadruple in quantity every 20 hours,which no other plant on earth can do. Know for its growth factors called , Chlorella Growth factor or (CGF) which is responsible for its amazing growth stimulating properties. CGF is considered the healthiest substance known because it is the most powerful component of the most potent food in the world. Chlorella consists of 60% protein, 20% carbohydrates, contains good healthy fats, amino acids, amino peptides, gycoproteins, B-Complex vitamins,minerals, phyto-hormones, polysaccharides, growth factors, RNA, DNA, and substances that are not found in other food sources known, WOW ! A good source of Chlorella comes from the company "Sun Chlorella" they also sell a liquid version that's very potent and expensive called "Sun Wakasa Gold Plus" look into it, you won't regret it ! Chlorella is truly a "Super Food".

Spirulina – A blue-green algae that commonly grows in fresh lakes and ponds , is considered a complete protein source, as it contains a complete balance of amino acids and essential nutrients, epecially iron. Spirulina powder is also more readily consumed much easier on the digestive system than regular protein sources like red meats. This nutrient dense super food is now being considered and discussed as a natural sustainable food source with the potential to end world hunger. With its high protein content of 61 to 71% with all of its essential amino acids in complete balance, and is one of the only plant sources to contain a significant amount of vitamin B12. This is another super food that time just doesn't allow for the scope of this book, but bares looking into. In essence it embodies the simplest form of life.

Acia Berries – A delicious fruit that is native to South America and is about the same size as a blue berry , that's considered one the world's super foods. It is very nutrient dense fruit that has generated quite amount of attention here in the US. Acia Berries have 10 times the amount of anti-oxidants than red grapes or red wine,rich in essential fatty acids, and is also a good source of fiber. Loaded with natural enzymes and cofactor's for digestion and nutrient absorption. Acia also contains Phytosterols, hormones with several health benefits, amino acids, and provides all the vital vitamins and important minerals.

Wheat Grass Powder - This is a product obtained from dehydrating the extracted juice from wheat grass and sold as a dietary supplement. Wheat Grass is valued for its high nutritional content of high levels of beta-carotene, amino acids, B-viatamins,fiber, and the enzymes. With its high chlorophyll content and substances with a pelthora of biological functions ranging from increasing hemoglobin production to improve fertility and to prevent hair from turning gray. Wheat Grass is also a good source of vitamin B12,vitamin C and iron.

Bee Pollen – Considered one of nature's most complete nourishing foods with a 40% protein content containing nearly all of the nutrients required by humans. Another interesting fact about bee pollen is that it can not be synthesized in a laboratory. Bee Pollen contains all of the essential components of life. The percentage of rejuvenating elements in bee pollen far exceeds those of other natural super foods. Bee Pollen corrects the deficient nutritional imbalances commonly found in those with nutritional deficiencies. Cultures throughout the world have used bee pollen as a restorative tonic and health aid. According to the researchers of the Institute of Apiculture,Taranov, Russia, "Honey Bee Pollen" is the richest source of vitamins found in Nature in a single food. Bee Pollen is a complete food and contains elements that products of animal origin do not possess . Contains more proteins than animal sources. It contains more amino acids than eggs,beef,and cheese. Is extremely rich in Rutin , and may have the highest content of Rutin than any other source,and it provides a high content of RNA and DNA.
Bee pollen comes in granules or powder that can be consumed right out of the jar,with a teaspoon dose being the right amount. It can be also added to cereals, protein shakes,and smoothies for a quick pick me up.

Pomegranate Juice – An ancient food that has symbolic meaning in many traditions and is mentioned throughout the old testament in the bible. Found in parts of the Mediterranean,India,and the Himalayan's, pomegranates are loaded with nutritional content that is particularly rich in vitamin-C, potassium, and B5 (pantothenic acid). Considered a powerful anti-oxidant that has incredible free radical scavenging affects that are just now being studied by scientists. Its powerful anti-oxidant effect makes pomegranate one natures richest source of free-radical scavenging anti-oxidants known today. In 2008, the Journal of Agriculture and Food Chemistry ranked pomegranate juice as one of nature's most healthiest fruit juices to drink.

Organic Cacao Powder – Cultivated in Mexico,South America and Central America for thousands of years that has been so highly valued by the native peoples once used its seeds as currency. The Aztec's believed it to be of a divine origin for health stimulating effect. By the 17th and early 18th centuries, chocolate was considered a cure for many illnesses and as well as a catalyst for provoking passion. Cacao powder is simply the cacao bean , that through a cold pressing process , has had the fat (cacao butter) removed. Cacao powder can be used to make chocolate by mixing it with cacao butter and a sweetener , Agave Nector is recommended.
Cacao has more anti-oxidant flavonoids than any other known food source tested so far.
It has up to four times the quantity of anti-oxidants found in green tea. Cacao promotes health cardiovascular function,protects you from metabolic toxins,increases your levels of specific neurotransmitters that help you feel good. Cacao beans are also rich in essential minerals such as magnesium and sulphur . It also contains a substantial amount of essential fatty acids , oleic acid , a heart friendly monounsaturated fat found also in olive oil, that may raise good cholesterol levels.
Note: to fully benefit from cacao's wide array of health producing affects, eat chocolate that is in its natural state as possible.
.

Colostrum Powder – Considered Mother Nature's best kept secret. Colostrum is the first lacteal secretion produced by the mammary glands of pregnant cow's. Its the first six hours after birth that is collected from birth that is valued in its pure state of natural colostrum. As the first food for new life, bovine colostrum is a natural immune-stimulant
that is fortified with natural growth factors,nutrients,vitamins,essential fats,enzymes,and minerals. Colostrum was carefully designed by nature as it was intended to sustain new born life. Taken by many athletes and bodybuilders for its growth enhancing effect,colostrum gives you a good source of insulin-growth-factor-1 (IgF-1) because it works!
Research has shown that colostrum is the one supplement that can bring help to everyone that uses it, largely because of its ability to perform many of the functions of human growth hormone (HGH) in the body. Colostrum has also been well documented in clinical observations that is supported by a large data base. Considered also the essence of pure nutrition that contains, immunoglobulins, growth factors, anti-bodies,vitamins,minerals,amino acids,enzymes,essential fats, and special other substances designed by nature to prime the body to face a life time of various micro-organisms and enviromental toxins. When purchasing colostrum make sure its from the first six hours of delivery and that its certified.

Raw Natural Unfiltered Honey – Raw unfiltered honey offers you a host of beneficial health benefits. From alleviating allergies to soothing sore throats. In actuality raw unfiltered honey is one sweet powerful remedy for all. For more than 3,000 years since it was farmed and used by the Egyptians, raw honey has always been considered the original super food. By providing health benefits beyond just basic nutrition like – providing a quick boost of energy,decreases muscle fatigue,soothes indigestion,soothes sore throats,rejuvenates skin conditions,soothes coughs, and acts as a preservative. Most of the commercial sold honey you find in grocery stores is of no nutritional value, devoid of nutrients that was heated and processed you should stay away from. Make sure your brand is raw unfiltered unheated pure honey, that is of nutritional value packed with natural enzymes,vitamins,minerals,and trace elements.

Final Thoughts - There you have it ! A list of super foods,supplements and additional information on some of the more beneficial nutrients that hopefully will help you to understand and gain some knowledge so that you can make better informed decisions when purchasing supplements concerning your cause. This was not the be-all to end-all to supplement guides or super foods, but which were in my opinion the ones I thought would benefit you much more effectively and nutritionally. So whether you are an avid competitor or a beginner that is starting out to change their physique, I hope you will have learned something of value that will help speed up your cause and provide great health to you in your quest !

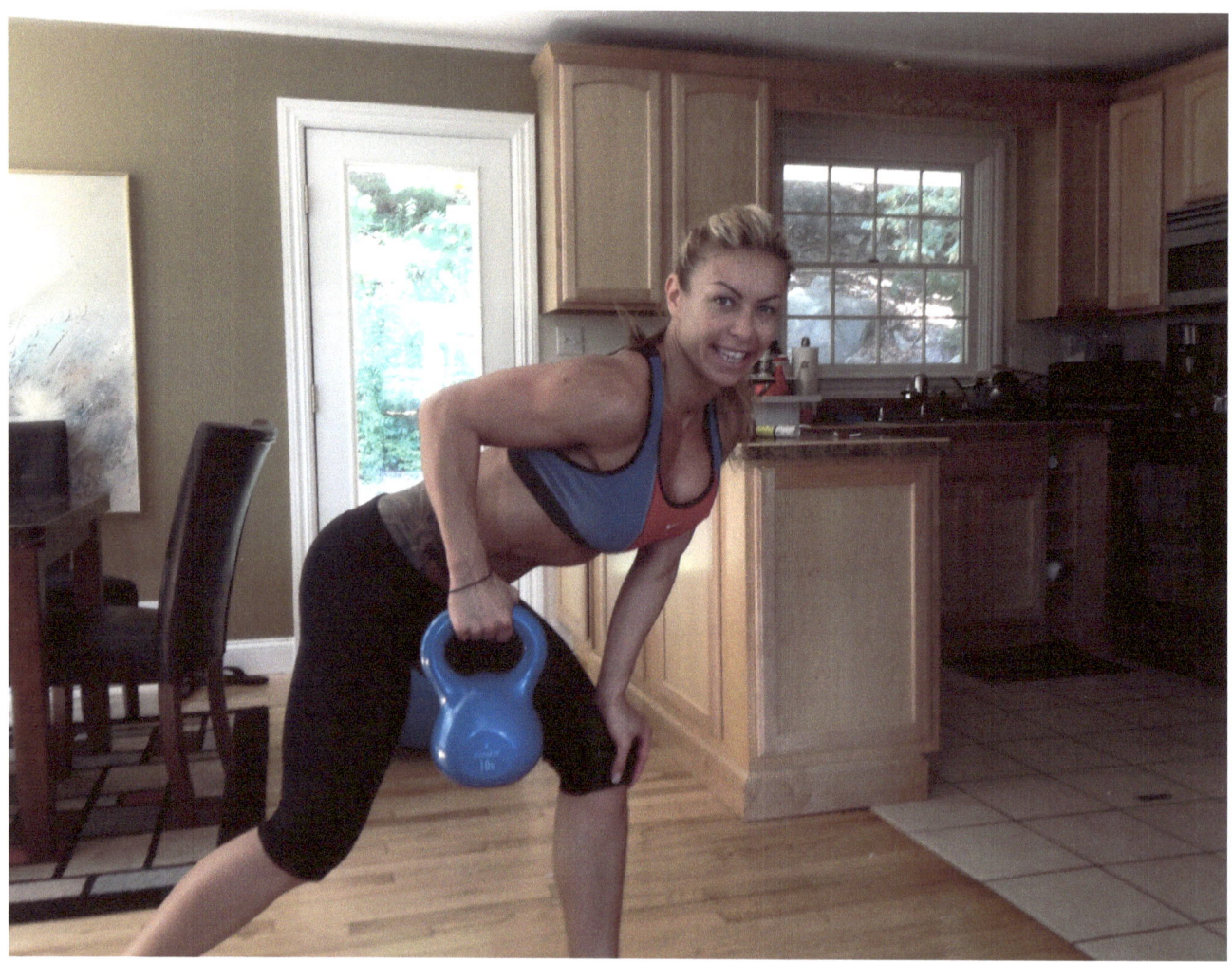

Chapter 8
Sugar and It's Harmful Affects on The Body
"The Cause of Obesity and Illness"

Consuming sugar right after exercise, your post-exercise window to muscle growth will have a significant negative impact on both of your insulin sensitivity and your human growth hormone (HGH) production. In addition, research shows that by consuming fructose, including that from fruit juices within this two hour window of post exercise nutrition will decimate your HGH production.

This shuts down your synergistic benefits of HGH that you've just stimulated through exercise negating the effects of your training. You gain the calorie burning affect but will not benefit from the induced muscle stimulating effect of HGH. This is a very important fact to always consider if you want maximum affect of muscle stimulation. Research teams have also demonstrated that carbohydrates are burned during exercise in direct purportion to intensity of training.

The fat burning affect is also correlated with intensity. However the actual fat burning affect does not take place till after the training session, during the recovery phase. By applying this synergy effect of the post-exercise two hour window, very important in maximizing the natural HGH stimulating effect that was just produced by high intensity training. For those older athletes forty and over that want the maximum induced benefit of exercise induced HGH,a very important point to remember.

These days carbohydrates are now being considered an evil cause to obesity and weight gain. However not all carbohydrates are considered bad, and are necessary foods needed by the body. But the most evident of these bad sugars are the refined carbohydrates that are used excessively in our daily diets, like pasta,white four products, bread, rice, sweets, chocolates, candies, and soft drinks.

The desired carbohydrates are the ones that have not been manipulated by humans that have produced industrially. The natural carbohydrates like fruits and vegetables are the preferred choice. But there are some with a very sweet flavor that are high in natural sugars such as fructose that can turn into body fat. Examples are bananas,raisins,and mangoes. Carbohydrates that are refined industrially have a molecule that is so small that the body quickly turns them into glucose with no effort at all. Also high starch foods such as bread,pasta,potatoes, break down into sugar that will stimulate the production of the neurotransmitter serotonin in the brain which is responsible for suppressing our appetite and regulating our moods.

Serotonin, once released into the blood stream produces a calming affect making you feel content and happy. It also reduces our pain threshold and can make us sleepy. Carbohydrates can be a powerful drug , and if it was bottled and patented it would be a scheduled drug. Sugar is along the same lines as common anti-depressants ,as they both help to release serotonin levels in the brain. When levels of serotonin drop, a gloomy feeling takes over and then the need for simple sugars take over.

The average American consumes over 150 lbs. Of sugar a year, and most of it comes from refined carbohydrates that is found everywhere. By the time most of us become aware that we are swimming in a sea of glucose, we are then seeing the physical effects of it. Illnesses like hypoglycemia, diabetes, candidiasis, and a suppressed immune system are all attributed from the effects of simple sugars. This is all a result of the constant battle to regulate your blood sugar as your body is constantly pumping out insulin to stop the over flow of sugar.

There is an economic reality that exists behind all of this. Popular name brand manufactures make most of their money off of producing carbohydrate products. Companies like "General Mills, General Foods, Quaker Oats, Nabisco,Kellog's, and Nestle" - almost all of their products are refined carbohydrates which are by far their biggest source of income for their food industry. Refined carbohydrates are big money makers and at the same time this is whats causing a wide spread epidemic on obesity and diabetes. The driving force behind all of this is money ! So the important and wise thing to do is, inquire some awareness and read the labels of products that we are purchasing, to protect ourselves and our loved one's.
Scientists today are now telling us that one out three children will develop diabetes in their lifetime. The good news is that this can be prevented by reading labels of consumer products at the grocery store, and we actually don't have to give up our sweet tooth, because there are alternatives. **Here is a**

list of some excellent sugar substitutes that you can use -

Agave Nectar - Sweeter than honey that has a very low glycemic index and is low in calories. Agave nectar is a combination of fructose and glucose that does not have an affect on blood sugar.the syrup blends in quickly in most hot and cold drinks, and can be used on pancakes and cereals.

Stevia - A natural herb that is an excellent and healthy substitute to use as a sugar alternative. Stevia is 300 times sweeter than regular table sugar with zero calories that doesn't cause spikes in blood sugar levels and is also very popular with those that have diabetes. Approximately one teaspoon of the calorie free stevia will substitute for a whole cup of regular white table sugar. Look for popular name brands of commercially sold stevia like - "Truvia" and
"PurVia".

Raw Natural Honey (unfiltered & unheated) - Considered a super food by many health experts. Raw unprocessed honey is loaded with anti-oxidants, amino acids, vitamins,enzymes and carbohydrates. Please note that processed honey is not the same as raw natural honey, processed honey is exactly that – processed ! stripped and devoid of all its natural nutritional value, that is basically no different than plain old table sugar.
Most of the honey found on shelves at the supermarket is processed honey that has been pasteurized and heated ,but if you look carefully you may be able to find raw unfiltered honey. Some types of honey like red clover or orange blossom, have a lower glycemic index, that dissolve more slowly into the blood stream and have a less effect on blood sugar levels. The best place to buy raw unfiltered honey is a natural health food store.

Xylitol – is a natural sugar alcohol sweetener found in the fiber of fruits and vegetables. Xylitol has a low glycemic index and is also low in calories and is considered a healthy sugar alternative for those with diabetes. Xylitol also helps fight cavities and is used as a common ingredient in most commercial chewing gums.

Maple Syrup – this is a naturally occuring sweetener that is an excellent sugar substitute for refined sugar, maple syrup is loaded with natural minerals, especially high in zinc and manganese.Maple syrup can help the body balance cholesterol levels.

Brown Rice Syrup - considered to be one of the healthiest natural sweeteners in the food industry since it is produced from a whole food source and is made up of simple sugars. For a bit of sweetness,brown rice syrup can added to toast,sweet potatoes,whole grains, or in tea.

The Worst Sugar Substitutes , Artificial Sweeteners

#1.Acesulfame K – aka "Sugar Twin"
#2.Aspartame - aka "Equal or Nutra Sweet"
#3.Sacchrin – aka "Sweet N' Low"

Note: Nutra Sweet is found in over 6,000 foods, including cereals,sugarless gum,and soda's. This sugar substitute has been scientifically proven to health problems in humans and animals such as Alzhiemer's, headaches,and cancer which are some of the known health problems associated with artificial sweeteners. In the 70's researchers noted that sacchrin caused cancer in laboratory rats, and adds to the body's overload of toxins. The chemicals found in sacchrin can cause inflammation,hormonal imbalances,diabetes, and heart disease.

Researchers at Purdue University found out that lab animals given foods sweetened with artificial sweeteners had gained more weight than those animals that had consumed just plain ordinary table sugar.

Organic Sugar – this typical widely used sugar is derived from sugar canes grown without chemicals or pesticides. It is typically darker in color than table sugar because it isn't processed to the degree that white table sugar is, and it also contains some molasses and retains a nutritional value.

Organic Palm Sugar – This is the next best thing to natural sweeteners. Palm Sugar is a nutrient rich ,low glycemic crystalline sweetener that tastes,and looks like regular table sugar, but is completely natural and unrefined. Palm sugar comes from the flowers growing high on top of the coconut trees which open to collect their rich liquid nectar. The nectar is then air dried to form a crystalline sugar thats naturally brown in color and rich in a number of key vitamins and nutrients, including minerals,phytonutrients, potassium,zinc,iron,and vitamins B1,B2,B3,and B6.
Palm sugar also has calories just like carbohydrates , but due to its extremely low glycemic index, its calories are absorbed into the blood stream at a significantly slower rate than regular refined table sugar. This natural alternative to natural sweeteners should be of importance to those that need to watch their blood sugar levels.

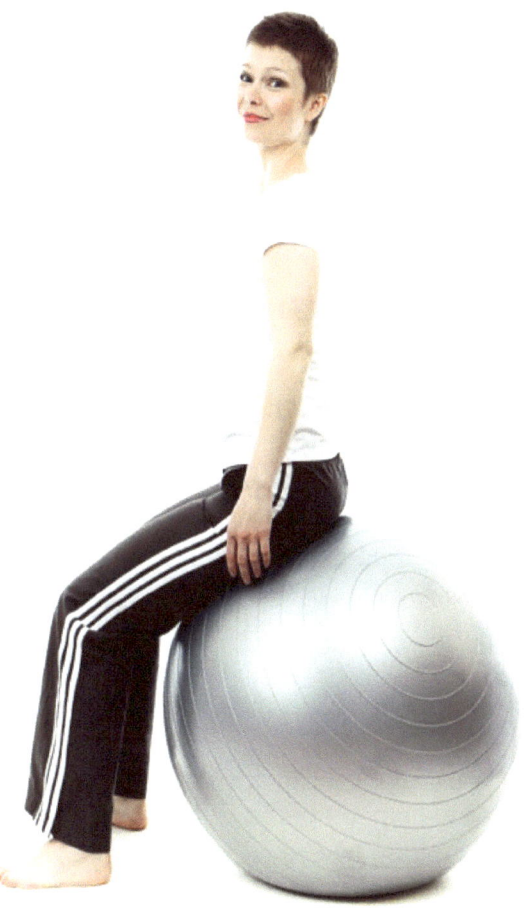

Chapter 9
Toning Your Buttocks & Getting Rid of Ugly Cellulite

A beautiful body starts with a sexy butt. Some women want the same muscle and toned behind as the top models that grace the cover of women's fitness magazines. 90% of women in America have some form of cellulite from their behind area down to their upper and lower thighs. Cellulite is the dimpling of the surface skin area found especially on your butt,stomach and thighs. This is caused by an uneven distribution of fat in between your skin and muscle tissue.

Women of all body types,fitness levels, and age have cellulite, but it is more common in older women and heavier women. You have to understand that even thin people also have a layer of fat under their their skin, because cellulite is a layer of fat separated by fibrous strands of connective tissue, which in turn pulls the skin down thus creating cellulite.

In this chapter we will eliminate all the confusion you have experienced in the past on trying to eliminate this ugly issue. We will simply things for you and by the end of this chapter you will have your own personal recipe for getting rid ugly cellulite issues.

Lets look at some of the contributing factors that cause cellulite -

    1) A lack of muscle tone due to lack of exercise.

    2) Poor micro-circulation,blood flow to the smaller areas of your lower body.

    3) A higher ratio of estrogen (fat storing hormone) to testosterone a (fat burning hormone) which could also be due to poor diet,age,or illness.

    4) Reduced collagen production (a skin tighting protein) due to poor dietary habits, lack of protein sources.

Actually all of these specified factors are basically inter-related. A lack of muscle tone due to muscle stagnation from not exercising will reduce your metabolic rate, which in turn make it harder to burn and metabolize the dimply fat stores just under the skin surface. Poor circulation also will make it difficult for the blood supply to reach and break down fatty acids, and the lower levels of testosterone make store fat. So by attacking all of these specified areas ,you will then make it easier in eliminating the cause of a dimple free cellulite condition.

The good news is that by using the specified exercise routine and techniques with a select dietary plan, you will have a program for that's been made custom tailored for your needs that you can use over again to deal with the root cause of cellulite. Weight loss programs do not get rid of cellulite or tone and shape your buttock area, a specified diet and exercise program will with a few added techniques including that will help you speed things up in this area that will allow you to have the body that you most desire.
This specified program will help you to increase the firmness of the muscles in your legs and butt, increase the tightness in your skin and help to optimize your hormone levels.

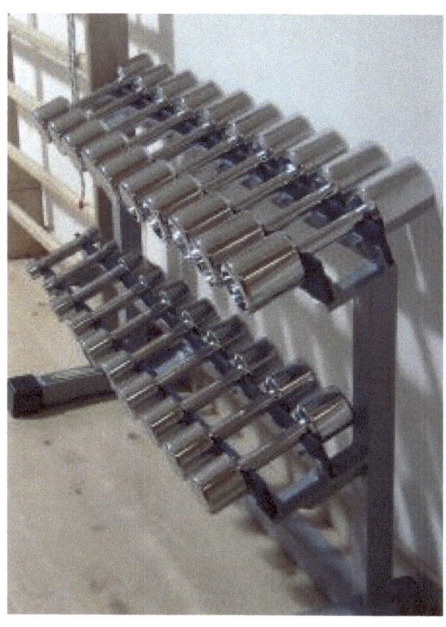

Chapter 10

Exercise Program For getting Rid of Cellulite and Toning Your Butt Putting It All Together

(1) **Eat a Natural Plant Diet** – by eating a natural plant-based diet, it can help you get rid of cellulite that much quicker,tone and shape your body, and lose some of the un wanted pounds. This also means you have to stay away from unhealthy processed foods that contain fats at the same time .try and consume as much fresh vegetables and fruits , and aim for atleast a 60% reduction in caloric intake or more.

If you need help in this area,i recommend you read the "80/10/10 Diet" by Graham Douglas. This book will give you a whole new outlook on nutrition.

(2) **Use other forms of supplementary techniques** to help you improve the

appearance of your skin. This includes massage and skin brushing techniques that

can become quite effective in stimulating blood flow to those trouble cellulite

areas. Use your basic massage oils mixed with pure lemon oil ,and apply it on as

massage and skin brush the areas associated with cellulite. By Brushing and

massaging, you will stimulate the lymphatic by removing toxins that were

trapped in fat stores and removing the dead skin cells by stimulating new ones.

<u>Note</u>: *Your diet basically needs to do only a couple of things – that is reduce your level of sugar intake, as this will help accelerate fat burning. Increase your circulation by stimulating blood flow to the problem areas with massage and skin brushing, this would be after your training,and take a cold shower as this would have a big and effective impact on blood circulation and hormonal response.(very Important)*

Exercise Routine Tailored For Buttock & Thigh Area

Cardio – this is done for 10-to 15 minutes to get your metabolism and blood flow going.

Exercise's – Your group of exercise's will be done in a circuit fashion meaning doing one after the other, without any rest in between. Once you finish all of them rest and then do them all over again.

This will stimulate a strong hormonal response and burn those extra calories.

Keep in mind that you should be doing these exercise for at least 2 to 3 sessions per week, but preferably 3 times a week done every other day for the best results possible.

Exercise Routine -

Squats – This exercise targets your buttocks very well and will help you build over all body strength. Do this with a barbell done with 50% of your max weight but do not sacrifice form. Make sure on the way down that your buttocks touch your ankles by going down as far as you can go, your feet should be spread apart about shoulder width.

Reps should be minimum of 10 reps, and don't forget you will be doing a circuit fashion as stated earlier. So we are not going to be concerned with sets here.

Lunges – This can be done with weights, dumbells held at your sides for extra resistance

Simply stand at an erect standing position and lunge forward with a leg quite far extending in front of you with your knee trailing towards the ground with your shin touching the floor. Then lift back up again and repeat it with the other leg. You can also walk around like this or just do it in one particular area. Don't forget as you go down while extending your leg to tighten or squeeze your buttock area. Your rep range should be 12 to 15 reps. Lunges are one the best exercises that will tone and shape your thighs and buttocks quickly and give you that desired look.

Cycling – this can be done on a stationary machine or several minutes while trying to increase the resistance as you get stronger. Cycling will help to tighten your buttock region as well as your back part of your thighs. Keep a rate of speed for a certain length of time while keeping the resistance going till finished.

Step-Ups – Stepping machines are very good for overall leg development and your buns. If your gym does not have a step up machine you can do this exercise with blocks by stepping up and down alternating each leg, you can also add resistance to this movement by hold a set of dumbells at your side.

Well, that's it as far as the exercise's go, which is basically the only amount that you will need, but remember the circuit fashion as we mentioned before, to be at least 2 to 3 circuits. With some light cardio done in the beginning of the first circuit.

Keep in mind that the butt is the largest and strongest muscle in the human body and these four exercise's will target the butt area like no other set of exercise's can. This is a short and effective workout that will get you the results that you've been looking for. Just doing two to three circuits of these set exercise's , you will begin to feel the burn in your thigh and buttock area.

Always remember to keep the resistance up and the intensity as you get stronger with each week, by adding an extra circuit fashion to your existing routine. You can take this to the next level as you progress further on with each passing week by adding weight to those specific exercise that are done with additional weight like with squats and dumbells.

Supplements To Add To Your Workout Program

- ⅄ **Glutathione-** this supplement will help support your immune system and recovery progress. Dosage should be 500 to 1,000 mgs two times aday.
- ⅄ **7-Keto DHEA -** was recently made popular by Dr.OZ as potentially the greatest belly fat reducing supplement that will help support your metabolism by stimulating your thyroid gland.
- ⅄ **Mega T Green Tea** – a natural weight loss aid that will help stimulate fast loss by boost your

metabolism and supplying your body with natural anti-oxidants.

- ⋏ **Vitamin/Mineral Supplement** – added insurance to supplement your diet by making sure adequate levels of nutrients are covered. Good choice is "All-One"

powder viamin/mineral formula with added anti-oxidants.

Closing Thoughts

What you have before you is a simple to follow routine that is not to demanding and taxing on the body, that basically be completed with easy leaving you with a ready made established program that has been tested and well received. I wish you well in your physical quest of health and fitness.

For more information on muscle,health & fitness, please feel free to see my online blog at http://tonyxhudo.wordpress.com/ or http://musclehealthandfitness.blog.com/